Yoga Poses

Benefits of Yoga Practice According to Yoga Sutras of Patanjali

Timothy Morrison

Table of Contents

Introduction

"36.7 million Americans or 15% of US adults practice yoga in the US"

- From the report by Yoga Alliance about yoga in the US 2016.

The United States medical practitioners, as well as chiropractors, are concerned about the increasing amount of traumas which individuals end up getting at yoga training, particularly by the "high-speed" type also known as "power yoga" which comes into play increasingly more into fashion in the last years. Just as professionals remember, right now there had not recently been a growth very similar to that ever since the Eighties while Jane Fonda started off to promote aerobic exercise.

A couple of years ago, «Boston Globe» correspondents presented instances of "victims" eagerness for yoga training. As a result, a thirty-year individual was looking for operation after he got his knee joint damaged. A lady with broad knowledge of yoga exercise injured the neck after practice with a whole new "guru." One other guy destroyed a nerve and as a consequence lost responsiveness of his thigh.

Given that professionals recognize, in many instances, yoga exercise is less dangerous compared to several other techniques. Nevertheless, lots of people misunderstand it, switching it into contests, and even without preparatory coaching as well as necessary information results into accidental injuries.

To have an understanding of the advantages of yoga exercise, it's vital that you realize that it's not only stretching out. Yoga is larger, even if you don't include any particular spiritual or religious part into your practice.

Stress reducing is the benefit with a good number of testimonies. However, given that stress is a huge element in just about all facets of your overall health. Stress elimination is a worthy reward.

Nature is organized in such a way that time always operates against the life. Certainly one of the situations associated with the local order is a simple fact, which ultimately this order is depleted. The instant an individual is born, the deflection of life-support processes is continually accumulating. Doing yoga exercise can a lot slow down the standard rate of the entropy process. Yoga certainly influences the activity of immune system. It's not just invigorating, but setting immunity work gently. It permits yoga practice to be evenly useful both at immunodeficiency and also at autoimmune disease problems.

Yoga exercise is a step-by-step activity revitalizing the motion of the system to the order of a greater level. At the particular phase of this scheme, the relationship between the individual and his systemic mind happens to be optimized.

F. Capra («Tao of physics», 1975) previously had looked into many cultures as well as customs attempting to explain basic rules of well-being and longevity. He came to the conclusion that you have just 2 of them. There was the overall flexibility of the backbone along with the ability to deep relaxation. Well, both these skills are available by yoga exercise.

Yoga is similar to the healthy nutrition. If you use it correctly in the optimal quantity, it will lead to unmatched physiological as well as psychological health. And this eventually reflects into your life, improving its overall quality. However, if you are probably trying to carry out the whole thing in yoga exercise instantly, the outcome could be comparable to striking random unusual postures.

It will be the motionless body along with the quiet mind (accomplished both in asana as well as in pauses between all of them) which is the fundamental factors for starting the technique of unprompted treatment of the system.

In daily life, the conscious mind is continually associated with the steps involved in socializing with the outside world and by no means stays vacant. This emptiness or silence of mind can solely take place in the performance of asana in line with Sutra 46, chapter II.

By some estimation, yoga in the USA is now a most dynamically developing form of physical activity. Here is the diagram which reflects that dynamic.

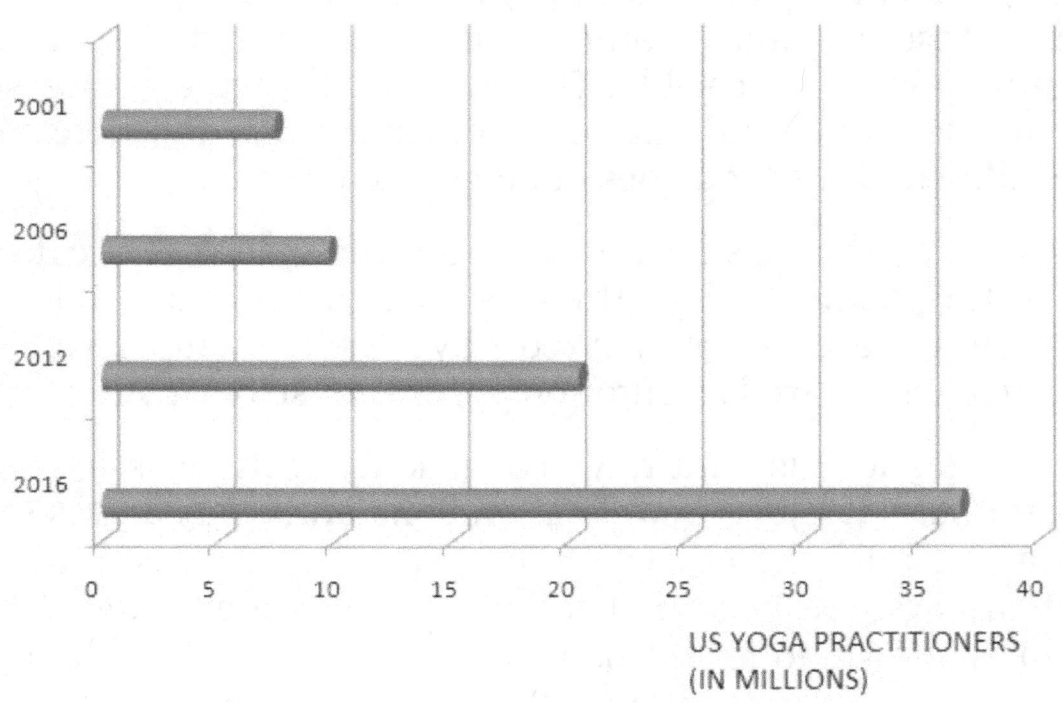

US YOGA PRACTITIONERS
(IN MILLIONS)

The approach of a person of the western mentality to yoga contains a drastic and rather dangerous mistake. Ancient texts do not mean the direct strong-willed control regarding the asana performance or meditation.

By its character, yoga is the ability of indirect control of the functional psychosomatic parameters (both controlled and automatic) using setting up specific conditions in both the entire body as well as the mind.

Definition of PSYCHOSOMATIC: of, relating to, concerned with, or involving both mind and body

We are going to look at the following instance. Eating is essential for surviving. Having acquired the cash, you can easily get the food, carry it home and even likely prepare it, arrange the table and sit down, get your hands on the food, put them into the mouth, gnaw and eat it. These would be your personal actions. However, what else could you do with the ingested food? Almost nothing, no more direct manipulations are feasible. The entire body further processes the meals alone, without your control. While the digestive breakdown of the food goes on, it gets to be self-regulating.

It is far from being smart to interrupt the means of breaking down the food. Through the existence of evolution, natural operations are characterized by their high level of effectiveness as well as autonomy from conscious control.

This instance is entirely congruent with classical or traditional yoga just as well. Yoga constantly was and is still the art of an indirect realignment. I only create conditions that my system by itself has led to the proper order. This order is known under the name of homeostasis. It is a hidden thing. We "learn" about its existence just after the appearance of disorder.

In traditional yoga, your body takes on asana, and the consciousness is virtually turned off not becoming involved with the process. The sequencing of poses, in the beginning, has no special meaning as it is defined according to the level of health and flexibility.

The irrelevant complication is not needed in yoga practice in any way. It is energy-consuming, dangerous, and not suitable for the proper yogic state of consciousness.

Classical Yoga Centers around Patanjali's Yoga Sutras.

"Asana is reached at the termination of effort or concentration on the infinite"

- «Yoga Sutras of Patanjali»

Sutras of Patanjali are a metaphorical explanation of the algorithm of traditional yoga practice. Such kind of yoga leads to the clearing and regeneration of your system. Then your contacts with outside world become optimal, as well as cooperation between your consciousness and sub-consciousness.

Sūtra (Sanskrit sū´tra), literally means a rope or thread that holds things together, and more metaphorically refers to an aphorism (or line, rule, formula), or a collection of such aphorisms in the form of a manual.

There are 196 Sutras of Patanjali. They are divided into eight 'limbs'. Practice on the physical level is only one of these parts. The name of this particular limb is asana. When you master your physical practice, you will be capable of learning other sides of yoga.

Patanjali is known as the father of yoga. He defines yoga as the cessation of recognition with the mental wandering. The first of Sutras is "Yoga is now." And this conception is not as simple as it sounds. Actually, achieving the now is challenging task.

Benefits of Yoga Practice

"The top 3 reasons people do yoga are the enjoyment of yoga itself, yoga's impact on health and yoga as a stress reliever"
- From the report by Yoga Alliance about yoga in the US 2016.

Practicing classical yoga always leads to recovery of the whole body system. That's why traditional yoga technique is a unique one. We consider such kind of yoga is a psychosomatic maintenance installed in the particular practice.

You could step by step rehab your physical and psychic health with the help of yoga. Of course, the result depends on your current stage and your age too. In theory, you could be regained from the weak position. But in real life, we always meet some difficulties. For instance, as a beginner, you need some adaptation period. Most likely, you will see results of practice only after that period.

Practice is a special "tempering" in the "fire" of yoga. When your body and your mind get ready, the siddhi appear.

Siddhi *(Sanskrit: siddhiḥ) is a Sanskrit word that literally means "perfection," "accomplishment," "attainment," or "success." It is also used as a term for spiritual power (or psychic ability).*

Rather than specifying their entire list, we will consider only one of them, "power." It is acquired only via long-term and quality practice of yoga.

We won't reside definition of every siddhi here. However, you should keep in your mind that any of these powers could be earned only by long-established and qualitative yoga practice.

There are too many variants how this power can influence practitioner's life. For example, you can notice that all issues you have met during nearest past are solved in the best of the possible way. Well, you should make a difference here. Your needs do not always coincide with your wishes. In fact, often they are opposite to each other. Your "power" doesn't support every dream generated by your mind.

You don't need too much time to get benefits of yoga poses. Yoga is an especial practice scheduled as part of your day which helps you to provide a high-grade life. Mentioned above power also impacts on relations with your family, friends, colleagues. The practicing person isn't in need of any sort of support anymore. It's opposite situation now. You become a source of calmness and energy for all people around you.

When you achieve some level of inner peace, you may notice that the favorable outcome in any affair relies solely on the quality of your calmness. Probably, you have already heard about benefits of brain work in alpha rhythm. So, throughout your practice, you are in alpha rhythm mostly.

Usually, your internal power directs situation in a right way even if the prognosis was adverse.

Traditional yoga improves the well-being of any person appreciably. If you are naturally healthy and well balanced emotionally, you still should practice gaining additional benefits and new opportunities.

General Guidelines

It is very special and positive ritual when you have woken up early in the morning then take your place on the mat and start practice. At some point in time, you start to feel your body entirely. You become a whole with your body, which bends and flows itself. All it happens without opposing, but with some primal pleasure. The ordinal thinking process is substituted by the inner silence, the rest, and the clarity. You get a positive impulse, and you keep it through the whole day long. You feel happy without particular reasons. You do not feel weariness, anxiety, irritation. You could build everything, to what you are capable on the base of your inner power.

The best time for yoga is precisely in the morning. If possible, don't postpone your practice to the evening.

Despite the similarity of all people, each one of us has his age, anthropometrical indicators, and health status. Certainly, you have also your natural level of flexibility. Due to a proper yoga practice, you can reach your limit, but it has never been the purpose of yoga. Yoga is not about development your acrobatic abilities. The value of the practice is something bigger. There is something like freedom from your mental vanity.

Thus, all-inclusive yoga recipe doesn't exist. You should master your practice personally individually. Your persistent attempts to force the body to complicated poses performing will result in injuries and regress in practice. So, the presence of experienced instructor is strongly recommended.

As a beginner you will probably go through the next several levels:

- Physical and psychological adaptation;

- Mastering a deep mental and physical relaxation;

- Creating an effective regimen of self-adjustment;

- Trying on advanced poses and techniques;

There should not be any discomfort during entering, holding, or exiting asana. It's a cornerstone of classical yoga. With the relaxation of your body and mind, all sensations pass out of sight. The intensity of practice remains within the typical range of routine activities, like walking, cleaning house, working on the computer, etc.

How actually should beginner execute an asana in a physical part? You should simply do asana. Just do it without impatience, or an expectation of result or excessive aspiration to make better, without any desire to do as in the picture.

To relax all muscles, you should run through the whole body with your attention. However, Sutras tell us just about the concentration on the infinity. So, how can you do that? The focus on the infinity means merely disengagement, not thinking about anything. And your inner silence is possible in deep relaxation of both mind and body.

To kick things off, when it comes to yoga as long as doing this will not affect your pose, shut your eyes. Seeing your surroundings while practicing is not OK. Closing your eyes has the added benefit of allowing you to avoid focusing on external things around you, which can aid in preventing you from concentrating on the senses. These static poses are used exactly for that very reason in order to release consciousness from the ordinary "contents."

When this is achieved, the solution has been found. The focus is solely on the body and not anything external, so there should be nothing binding or distracting you.

Asana

Mastering in asana means that your consciousness falls and the mental process becomes rarer. Along with this, the body starts to sink spontaneously in the form, "flowing down" to its absolute for today limit of flexibility.

You see, you should not do asana. You should simply be in asana! But the real comprehension of this trick and its implementation may cost a lot of time and efforts.

Performing asana correctly means to do so without any deception in you, or excessive diligence, and desire. Your will cannot change base properties of psychosomatics and processes in life support system.

For those who are just beginning, time of being in asana is mattered. It's an individual factor. There are signs in the body and mind that will tell you when to exit asana. Once you begin to feel these odd or uncomfortable sensations, you should immediately exit asana to avoid harming or injuring yourself. If you feel discomfort, or any abnormal sensations the moment you enter asana, this is a sign that your pose is too difficult for your expertise (or lack thereof) and that you should choose a more comfortable one. Unusual sensations can also be a sign that you have some possible injury or mental blockage making itself known.

Stretching asana may be repeated thrice in a row. If you are doing everything correctly, your body will effortlessly bend to the level attained the previous time and will continue to "flow" to a new provisional limit. Contrarily, if you find yourself struggling to hold poses, you most likely have some sort of unconscious mental blockage preventing you from advancing, or you have reached your current physical limitations of body's flexibility.

Other signals to exit emanate from the circulatory system, where you may experience burning, heavy breathing, numbness, and swelling during some positions. You may also experience pulsation in some areas of your body. If pulsation occurs in the same areas during different poses, then it may be a sign that you are injuring some blood vessels, or it is a symptom of underlying circulatory issues that you were unaware of.

Your exit from asana should be calm, flowing, without sensations and at ease, mentally and physically. To exit properly, allow your body to loosen naturally, almost straightening in the way a stress ball would after you squeeze it. If you any discomfort after exiting asana, pause and let it discontinue before entering the next posture.

When you perform the pose, make sure to hold it for the proper amount of time, so your body gets the maximum benefit from it. When you begin to feel certain symptoms and sensations, it is an indication that you should end or switch postures.

One vital part of asana is to remember that hurting yourself is contradictory to ahimsa. The fundamental principle of the classical yoga is a not producing damage to the own body. Pain is a signal of injury, so you should avoid pain.

After some practice in asana, you will keep to a minimum the number of muscles involved as well as the intensity of their work. The valuable exposure time in asana lasts from the moment when you are motionless until the coming of sensations. When you begin to feel these sensations, stop the asana.

You should not feel discomfort during asana. You should not sweat heavily; feel pain, or any other unusual sensations. The foundation of yoga is not to hurry, but to relax in a way that one cannot in daily life. Asana requires a particular state of mind as well, and it is very much a holistic process, though you may not notice this at first.

Yoga requires holding certain poses; in fact, this is the foundation of yoga. It is using your body's weight and parts; it is the moving and crossing of limbs, and changing the body so that you maximize benefits received from gravity.

Tough poses should only be done by those who can do them without exerting too much effort, both physical and mental. You should be able to maintain a relaxed state of mind while doing asana.

For those just beginning yoga, the first step is to direct one's gaze towards the body. The eyes are typically the easiest way in which you can focus. Eyes should remain closed during practice since almost everyone receives information visually and visual stimulation can great affect your ability to relax the mind significantly. With closed eyelids the eyeballs habitually keep reflex moving around or shaking.

Shavasana is the recommended choice for beginners, one should be able to relax the eyeballs in such a way that they no longer spontaneously move or twitch at random. Oftentimes the eyes will move to find the most comfortable position. The eye orbits start to perceive weight, occasionally lukewarm, and the mind relaxed sets on this sector. However, the moment something catches the attention of the eye, it will strain again and move around like they normally do. This is why it is important that one practice relaxing the eyes so that the mind can relax as well and the mental activity slows down.

After accomplishing total relaxation of muscles in asana, the human body does only work that is needed. If you avoid making your posture better despite the negative sensations, there is no risk of having traumas.

These descriptions will be applicable only for those people whose natural flexibility allows to perform all that poses rather freely. It is not worth even reading of these descriptions in the initial phase of mastering yoga for those who are capable of reproducing the form of asana only approximately. What sense does it make if the body is able to be bent in a position far from being similar to what is in the image? As the novice gets more practice and begins to grasp the technique, his body flexibility starts to grow in itself. The asana which did not resemble the original become to get more and more similar to that which is in the image. After this, texts can now be used as a form of guidance to the practice.

Corpse Pose (Savasana)

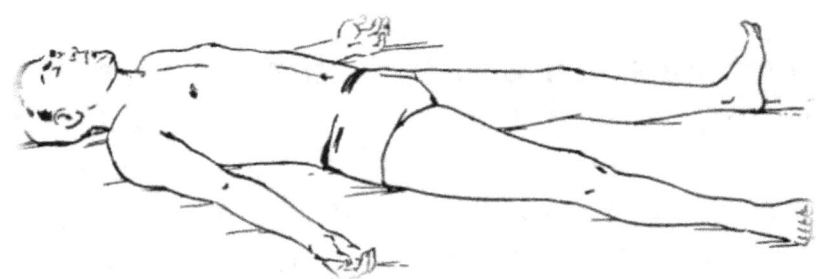

Bend your knees and sit on the floor, put both feet on the floor and recline backward on your forearms. Breathe in, then stretch the right leg slowly, do the same to the left leg pushing through the heels. Now both legs should be released with the groins softened. Ensure the legs are positioned at angles that are equal about the middle line of the torso. Also, take great care that both feet are turned out the same way. Now, the front pelvis should be narrowed, and the lower back should be softened but not flattened.

Reach for the ceiling with your arms perpendicular to the flooring. Oscillate gently from left to right, and then release your arms to the floor. Your arms should then be at angles that are equal about the middle of your body. Hands should be turned outwards.

Savasana serves the dual purpose of quieting the sense organ and the physical body. The wings of the nose, root of the tongue, channels of the inner ears and the bridge of the nose, which is between the eyebrows, should be softened. Release your eyes to the back of the head.

This pose should be maintained for at least 5 minutes for every half-hour of practice. To exit this pose, you should roll to one side (your right preferably) while exhaling once. Then two or three breaths should be taken. Your hands should press against your floor, and your body should be lifted.

If the relaxation is indeed profound, there is possible a little quivering of the muscle felt in Shavasana. This quivering seems like ripples of water. Usually, it starts on the left of the face if you are right handed. This quivering then extends to the right part of the body. It may then lead to a spontaneous dance of the muscles. This appearance is one of the ways by which mental stress is relieved, so there is nothing to fear or react.

Seated Forward Bend (Paschimottanasana)

Asana should always be done like breathing or walking. There should be no endeavor made to make them better. If no sensation is felt, then the asana is done perfectly.

Therefore, Paschimottanasana can be held for a long time. The body will jack-knife, and the torso will lie flat on straightened legs. This position won't give you any sensations which will be similar to Shavasana. You might feel tiny echoes of musculoskeletal movements, but they won't disturb the calmness of your mind.

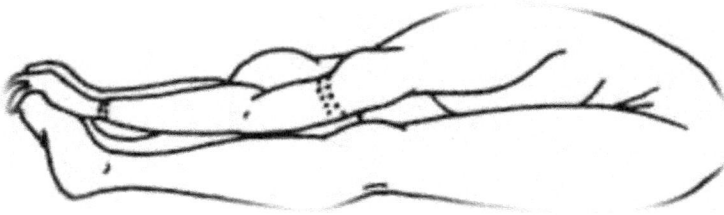

Support your buttocks on a blanket that is folded while you are seated with your legs in front of you. Your heels should be used to press actively. The top thighs should be pulled in a little, and then pushed to the ground. Your palms should then be pressed to the floor beside the hips, and the top part of the sternum should be lifted to the roof as the top thighs are brought down.

If you can, use your hands to take the side of your feet with your thumbs on the soles of your feet and your elbows fully extended. But if this is not possible, then you can loop a strap around the soles of your foot while holding the strap firmly.

When you wish to go further, don't use force to pull yourself into a forward bend. You should always lengthen the front torso into that pose while keeping your head raised. If your feet are being held, your elbows should be bent to the sides and lifted away from the floor. If the strap is being held, then your grip should be lightened, and your hands should be walked forward while your arms should be kept long.

As you inhale, you should lift and lengthen your front torso a little. As you make each exhalation, you should release a bit more into the forward bend. This way, the body oscillates, lengthens a little with the every breath.

This pose should be maintained for about one to three minutes. In order to come up, you should lift your torso away from your thighs.

Never try to force yourself into a forward bend especially when you are sitting on the floor. When coming forward, as soon as the space between your navel and pubis is shortening, you should stop, lift up slightly and lengthen again. At first, because you have tightness in the back of your legs, your forward bend will not go far forward and might look like sitting straight up.

Cobra Pose (Bhujangasana)

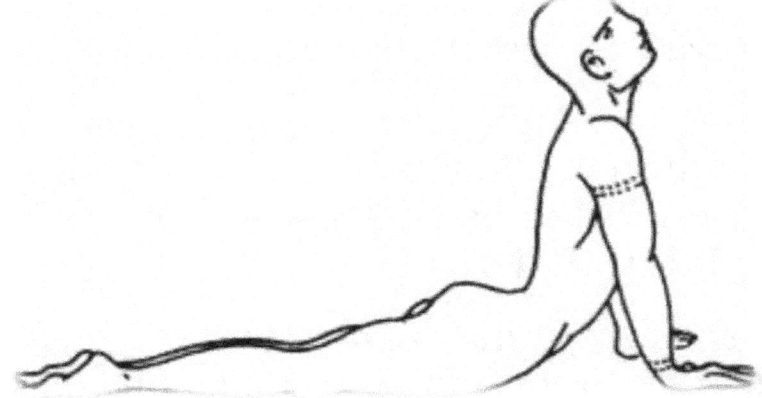

Lie on your tummy. Straighten your legs back and place the tips of your feet on the floor. Your hands spread out under your shoulders while your elbows are embraced into your body.

Your thighs, pubis and the tips of your feet should be pressed firmly to the ground.

Breathe in and then gradually straighten out your hands to lift your chest off the floor. Ensuring that you do not go beyond the height within which you can maintain a link with your pubis and legs. The tailbone should be pressed towards the pubis while the pubis itself is lifted towards the direction of the navel. Ensure the hip points are contracted firmly but not too much to avoid it toughening the backsides

Place the shoulder blades firmly against the back, pushing out the side ribs forward. Lift the shoulder blades through the top of the sternum while ensuring that the forefront ribs are not pushed forward. This way you prevent it from hardening the lower back region. Share the backbend equally all through the whole spine.

Maintain this posture for about 15 to 30 seconds, breathing effortlessly. Breathe out and discharge the back to the floor. Try not to do the backbend excessively. To discover the limit at which you can easily work without straining your back, release your hand from the floor for a split second so the height you will see will be the accurate extension you can comfortably work

Locust Pose (Salabhasana)

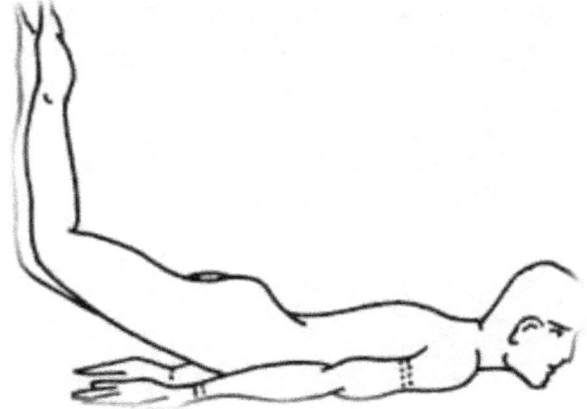

This pose might require you to cushion the floor beneath your pelvis and ribs with a blanket. After the padding, you then lie on your stomach while keeping your hands on the sides of your torso, with your palms raised up while your forehead remains on the floor. Place your big toes to face each other so that they can internally pivot your thighs, firmly place your backside so that your coccyx is pressed toward your pubis.

Breathe out and lift your head, upper middle, hands, and legs from the floor. Then, you rest on your lower ribs, stomach, and front pelvis. Place your backside firmly and try to reach through to your legs, starting from the heels to stretch the back legs, then through the bases of the big toes. Ensure the big toes are turned in the direction of each other.

Keep your arm raised parallel to the floor and extend back actually using your fingertips. Envision there's weight pushing down on the backs of the upper arms, and push up toward the roof against this opposition. Keep your scapulas pressed solidly into your back.

Look forward or somewhat upward, being mindful so as not to bulge your chin forward and crux the back of your neck. Ensure the base end of the skull is lifted while the back of the neck is kept long.

Maintain this posture about 30 to 60 seconds and then breath out and discharge at the same time. Breathe in and out a couple of time and try to repeat these 1 or 2 times if you wish. Starters often find it a bit challenging to lift the torso and the legs in this posture. Start the pose with your hands lying on the floor, a somehow back from the shoulders, nearer to your waist. Breathe in and gradually push your hands against the floor to help lift the upper middle. At that point, keep the hands set up as you do the posture, or after a couple of breaths, once you have ensured the chest is lifted up, swing them once more into the position explained above. Concerning the legs, you can practice the pose with the legs raised off the floor one at a time. For instance, you have to lift the left leg off the floor for about half a minute and then do same for the right leg if you want to hold the pose for one minute.

Shoulder stand (Sarvangasana)

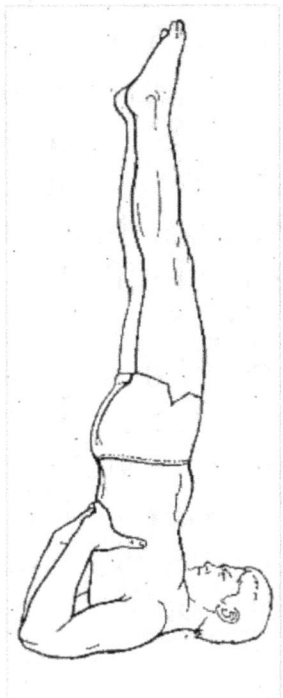

Lay down on your back, arms alongside your upper-body. Then bend your knees and put your feet on the floor with the heels close to the buttocks. Breathe out, press your arms firmly against the floor and lift your feet from the floor.

Keep your upper arms on the mat and stretch your palms against the reins. Raise your torso to the position relatively perpendicular to the floor.

Breathe in and bring your thighs in line with upper body keeping heels close to sitting bones. It's time now to unbend your knees.

To exit from the pose, breathe out and bend your knees again. Then roll your back down into the ground. Be careful and keep your head on the floor all the time.

Start with 30 seconds holding this asana. Add 5 or 10 seconds every time you practicing. Soon you will be able to stay for 3 minutes in Sarvangasana without any discomfort.

Plow Pose (Halasana)

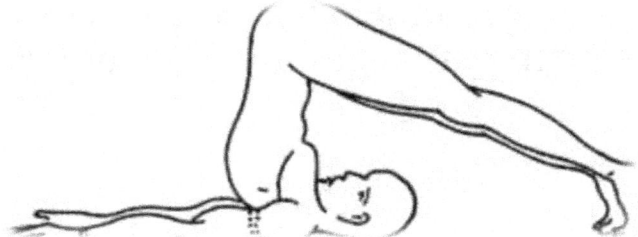

From Sarvangasana, breathe out and twist from the hip joints to gradually bring down your toes to the floor beneath and above your head. As much as you can, keep your middle region vertical and your legs completely straightened.

Keep your top thighs and tailbone raised toward the roof while your toes are kept on the floor. Draw your inward groins deep into the pelvis. Envisage that your middle region is dangling from the height of your crotches. Keep on bringing your chin far from your sternum and soften your throat.

You can keep on pressing your hands against the back of your middle region, while you press the back of your upper arm down. As another variant, you can discharge your hands from your back and straighten arms behind you on the floor, opposite the legs. Clip the hands and press the arms down on the support as you lift the thighs toward the roof.

Halasana is performed after Sarvangasana within 1 to 5 minutes. To release yourself from the pose, bring your hands back to your back once more, lift once again into Sarvangasana while breathing out, then move down to your back. In this particular pose, there is a possibility of you overstretching the neck by pulling the shoulders too far from the ears. In as much as the shoulder tops ought to push down into the support, they should also be lifted marginally toward the ears to hold the back of the neck and throat. You should open the sternum by keeping the shoulder blades firm against the back.

Bow Pose (Dhanurasana)

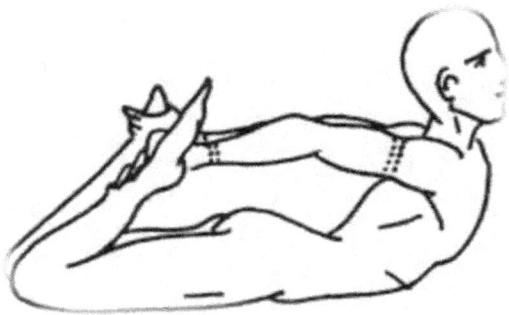

Lie on your tummy with your hands along your body and your palms placed up. Breathe out and flex your knees, bringing your heels as close as you can to your back side. Grab your lower legs using your hands through the back. Note that it must not be tops of your feet. Ensure your knees are not much wider than the breadth of your hips and keep your knees hip width throughout the period of this pose.

Breathe in and firmly lift your heels from your bottom and in the meantime, lift your thighs from the floor. This action will have the impact of pulling your upper torso and your head away from the floor. Tunnel the tailbone down toward the floor, and hold your back muscles soft. Keep lifting the heels and the thighs higher, while keeping the shoulder blades pressed against your back to be able to open your heart. Maintain the shoulder tops drawn away from your ears and look ahead.

Press your stomach against the floor. This act will make breathing to be difficult. However, you have to keep breathing and breathe more into the back of your torso. You do not have to stop breathing.

Maintain this pose for about 20-30 seconds. Free yourself gradually as you breathe out and breathe for a couple of times while you are rest.

Feel free to repeat this pose for 1 or 2 times more if you wish.

Hero Pose (Virasana)

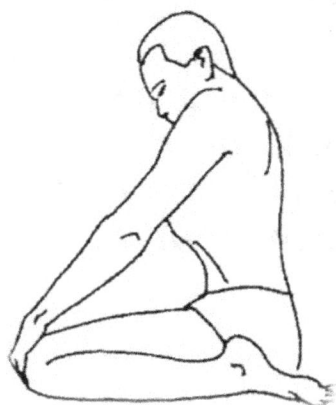

Go down on your knees on the ground and use the blanket as support between your calves and thighs if needed. Ensure your thighs are kept at an angle of 90° to the floor, and your inner knees are touching each other. Keep your feet separated from each other, a little bit wider than the knees and the tops of the feet should be kept flat on the ground. Then, you keep your big toes to face each other inwards while pressing the tops of both legs evenly on the ground.

Breathe out and sit midway, with your upper body kept a bit forward. Then, try sitting in between your feet.

Place a thick book or block in between the legs and use them to raise your buttocks if they do not comfortably rest on the floor. Keep a space of about the width of the thumbs between the inner heels and the outer hips. Press the heads of the thigh bones into the ground with your palms. Then keep your hands in your laps with palms down.

Place your shoulder blades strongly against the back ribs and straight your torso, like a fighter proud of his victories. Pull your collarbones slightly down and backward. Discharge the shoulder blades far from the ears. Protract the tailbone into the floor to hold the back-middle region of your body.

Initially, remain in this pose for about 30-60 seconds. Elongate your stay bit by bit up to 5 minutes. To release yourself, press your hands into the floor and raise your backside up a bit above the heels. Keep your ankles crossed underneath and sit backward on the feet and the ground. Then extend your legs before you. It might feel great to skip your knees here and there a couple of times on the floor.

Boat Pose (Navasana)

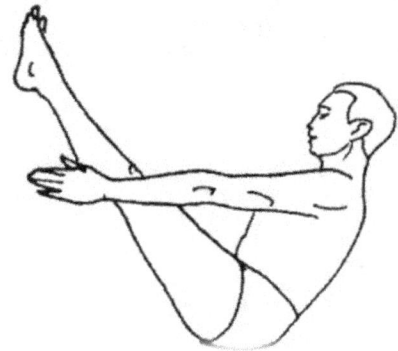

Take sit-on-the-floor with your legs straight before you and keep your hands firmly on the ground somewhat behind your hips with the fingers pointing towards the feet. Then lean back slightly. Make sure your back does not round as you do this. Sit on the "support" of your two sitting bones and tailbone.

Breathe out and twist your knees, then try raising your feet off the ground, so that the thighs are at an angle of about 45-50 degrees to the floor. Protract your tailbone into the floor and lift your pubis toward your navel. Gradually straighten your knees where possible, lifting the tips of your toes a bit over the level of your eyes. However, remain with your knees bent if this is not feasible maybe just lifting the shins parallel to the floor.

Straight out your arms parallel to each other and the floor. If it isn't feasible, you can place the hands on the ground near your hips, or otherwise, you hold on to the back of the thighs.

In as much as your abdomen should be kept firm, it should not be allowed to get hard and thick. It should be kept as flat as possible. Breathe effortlessly. Initially, you can remain in this position for about 10-20 seconds. Step by step you should increases the duration of stay to 1 minute.

Discharge the legs with an exhalation and sit upright while you inhale. You can rehearse this posture occasionally throughout your day even while sitting on your seat.

Downward-Facing Dog (Adho Mukha Svanasana)

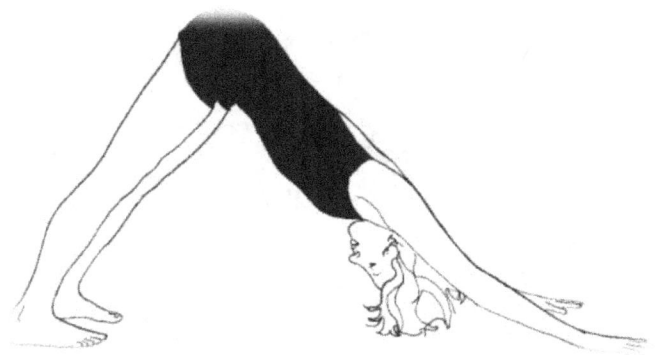

Get to the floor on your hands and knees. Your knees should be kept directly below your hips with your hands placed slightly onwards on your shoulders. Spread out your palms with your fingers turned out. Keep your toes under.

Breathe out and raise your knees above the ground. Initially, let the knees be kept bowed and the heels raised far from the floor. Then lift the sitting bones toward the roof. Breath out again and push your top thighs back and straighten your heels onto or down toward the floor. Straight out your legs.

Place your shoulder blades firmly against your back, then them wider and draw them toward the tailbone. Ensure the head is kept between the upper arms; never allow it to hang.

To come out, bend your knees to the floor while breathing out and rest.

Chair Pose (Utkatasana)

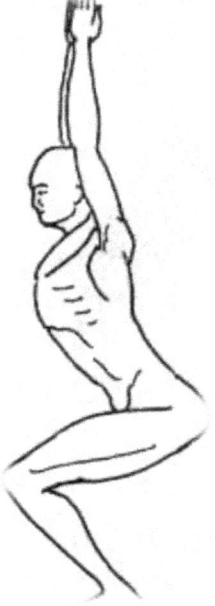

Stand with your feet together. Breathe in and raise your arms vertical to the ground. You can either join the palms or keep the arms parallel while the hands face inward.

Breathe out and bend your knees. You should keep your thighs as parallel to the floor as possible. Lean your upper body slightly forth until it stays at 90 degrees with the tops of the thighs. Ensure the inner thighs are parallel to each other and keep the heads of the thigh bones pressed toward the heels.

Maintain this position for about 30-60 seconds. To release yourself from this pose, make your legs straight while breathing in. Then breathe out and bring your arms back to your sides into the start position.

Eagle Pose (Garudasana)

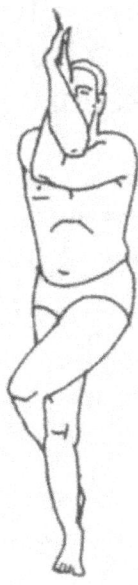

Stand with your feet together and with your knees bent slightly. Rise up your left foot and keep yourself balanced on the right foot. Then, you cross your left thigh over the right. Place your left toes pointed to the ground and kept the foot pressed back. After which you hook the top of the foot at the back of the lower right calf.

Straight out your arms. Then cross them in front of your torso in such a way that the right arm is kept above the left and then bend your elbows. Place the right elbow inside the crook of the left and maintain the forearm lifted vertically to the floor. Ensure that the back of your hands is facing each other.

Place your palms together. Ensure that the biggest finger of the right hand is passed in front of the little finger of the left hand and press the palms together as firmly as you can. Raise your elbows up and straight your fingers out to face the roof.

Maintain this position for about 15 to 30 seconds and release the legs and the arms and then stand in the start position. Go through the same process within the same time frame but your legs and arms inverted this time. As a beginner, you might have some difficulty to hook the lifted left leg behind the standing leg calf and keep it balanced on the standing foot.

For the first times, you might cross the legs and press the big toe of the leg foot instead of hook it. Keep the big toe pressed against the floor to help you hold it in balance.

Extended Side Angle (Utthi Parsvakonasana)

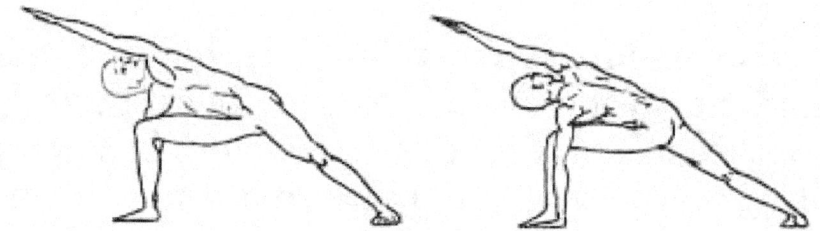

Stand with your feet to about 3.5 to 4 feet apart. Lift your arms parallel to the floor and let them be reached out actively to the sides. Your scapulas should be placed wide, and your palms kept down. Place the left of your foot a bit at a right angle to the right of your foot.

Keep the right heel aligned with the left heel. Roll the left hip slightly forth, toward the right, but rotate your upper body back to the left side.

Breathe out and curve the right knee in such a way the shin is placed vertically to the floor. You should bring the right thigh to be parallel to the ground.

Straighten out your left arm to face the ceiling and then twist your left palm in such a way that it will face towards the direction of your head. Then breathe in and reach the arm over the back of your left ear with your palm down. Redirect your head to face your left arm and discharge your right shoulder far from your ear.

Breathe out as you keep your left heel placed to the ground and lay your right upper body down as close as possible to the top of the right thigh. Keep your palms pressed on the ground just outside of your right foot.

Maintain this position for about 30-60 seconds and breathe in to come up. Most beginners often experience two challenges in this asana.

One of the problems is their inability to keep the back of their heels firm to the ground as they bend their front knee into this pose. The solution to this problem is to support your back heel against a wall. Imagine that you are pushing the wall away from you with your heel.

The other one is that they find it difficult to touch the fingertips of the lower hand once they are in this position. The solution for you is to rest your forearm on the top of the bent knee instead of trying to touch the ground.

Tree Pose (Vrksasana)

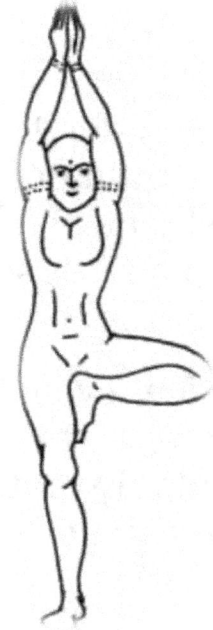

Stand with your feet together. Transfer your weight a bit more on the left foot and keep the inner side of your foot placed firmly on the floor and twisted your right knee. Use your right hand to reach out and hold your right ankle.

Your foot should be drawn up and placed the sole against the inner left thigh. Point your toes towards the floor and hold the right heel into the inner left groin. Clasp your palms together at heart.

Maintain this position for about 30-60 seconds. Breathe out and stand in the start position. Do the same asana within the same frame of time but with your legs reversed.

Conclusion

A lot of beginners fail to understand that total absence of something could be more valuable than its presence. This one is a primary reason why most of the novices overdo their asana practice, giving room to sensations of little pains which makes them feel that they are doing useful work.

During every asana practice, even at intermissions between them, we delegate powers to the system, to change and control the course of events. Everything else, such as feeling better, improved flexibility, relief of stress is results of this delegation.

'Action by not action' as described by Patanjali is the central principle of classical yoga. Traditional yoga is a gentle management of initial conditions. As a result, the system works in itself in a direction useful to it and hence helpful to me. Any physical or mental activity constructed from the beginning to the end on personal efforts and self-control is not classical yoga!

Combining mental silence with asana practice is partly a meditation, with all the effects flowing from it. The word 'partly' is used because for you to meditate you need not to move for an extended period which is impossible in most of the yoga poses.

We have already mentioned study 2016 about yoga in the US earlier in this book. There are few curious stats, which I would like to comment.

1.   There are almost 14 million yoga practitioners over the age of 50 in the US.

This one looks like pretty good evidence of positive impact of yoga practice on your active longevity. And it is worthy, isn't it?

2.   75% of yoga practitioners also engage in other physical exercises including running, group sports, weightlifting, and cycling.

Yoga teachers are seven times more likely to practice martial arts than is the average US adult.

As you can see, yoga is only a part of the physical culture for the biggest part of practitioners. Actually, I consider yoga practice as an excellent recovery from sports stress.

3.   98% of practitioners consider themselves to be beginner or intermediate level practitioners.

It was a key reason for writing this book. So, it is also a good cause to say one more time "thank you" for purchasing my book! I hope that you have enjoyed it. You should start your practice as soon as you can.

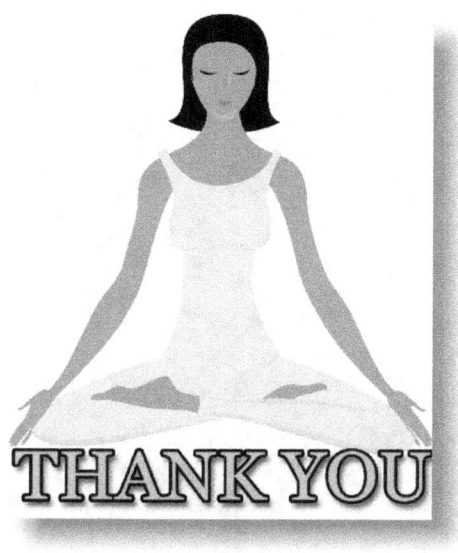